Bromelain

The active enzyme that helps us make the most of what we eat

Anthony J. Cichoke, D.C.

Keats Publishing, Inc. ▓ New Canaan, Connecticut

Acknowledgments
The author is extremely grateful to the following researchers and physicians for their excellent cooperation and insights: Drs. Karl Ransberger, Steven Taussig, Gerhard Stauder, Rudolf Inderst, J. Steffen, Peter Streichhan, J. Seifert, G. Gebert, Anthony Lopez, Wilhelm Glenk, Gert Klein, Michael W. Kleine, Sven Neu, Raul Ahumada, Heinrich Wrba, Otto Pecher and Tracey Mynott. A special thanks to Mrs. Karen Hood for her yeoman efforts. Further, I wish to thank Keats Publishing, Inc. for its never-ending faith and reinforcement. Finally, my deepest thanks to my wife, Margie, for her love and constant support.

Bromelain is not intended as medical advice. Its intention is solely informational and educational. Please consult a medical or health professional should the need for one be indicated.

BROMELAIN

ISBN: 0-87983-835-3

Printed in the United States of America

3 4 5 6   0 9

CONTENTS

In today's fast-paced society, we don't usually die from a caveman-type club to the head. Instead, we become ill, age and die because of chronic, degenerative disorders, such as heart disease, stroke or cancer. Our lifestyle, pollutants, food additives and preservatives, enzyme-dead fast foods, empty calories and stress wear down the body's resistance and kill us like a vicious thief in the night. These modern problems have literally sapped our bodies of needed enzymes and have caused modern diseases which are killing us before our time.

One way to improve health is by improving digestion. Eating fewer cooked foods and more enzyme-rich fresh fruits and vegetables can help your body to function better and give you increased energy.

Unfortunately, improving your diet might not be enough. Supplemental enzymes, such as bromelain, might be necessary.

This Good Health Guide will explain how bromelain, the enzyme found in pineapple, can improve your health by serving:

1. As a digestive aid to improve digestion and absorption of food nutrients;
2. As a systemic enzyme, working at the organ and cellular levels to fight inflammation and chronic disorders;
3. To improve absorption of medications, vitamins and other natural supplements;
4. Topically, to improve skin tone and also to debride devitalized tissue from burn injuries.

As mentioned, bromelain is an enzyme. Enzymes are catalysts that occur naturally in all living things. Every plant, microbe and animal must have enzymes. As catalysts, enzymes can speed up a reaction or help a reaction take place. All life processes consist (in part) of a complex series of reactions called metabolism. Enzymes produced naturally by the body are critical for metabolism, in fact, for all aspects of life. Without enzymes, life could not exist.

Enzymes are essential for the body to function. During digestion, enzymes are necessary in breaking down the proteins, carbohydrates and fats in our foods into smaller molecules for absorption. Other enzymes in the body are responsible for different functions, including respiration, growth, reproduction, vision, and the storage and release of energy. To date, about 3,000 enzymes have been identified in the human body.

Plants, too, use enzymes in their metabolism. To date, scientists aren't exactly sure of bromelain's role in the pineapple. It is possible that bromelain serves a protective role by interacting with other species, or it may defend against parasites or other pathogens. In his book, *Plant Proteolytic Enzymes*,[1] Michael Dalling states that proteases (such as bromelain) might serve to attract animals who would benefit the plant's reproduction. By eating the plants and seeds, the animals help disperse plant seeds over a wider area than would otherwise be possible.

Bromelain is a proteolytic enzyme. Proteolytic enzymes break up proteins into amino acids. Each enzyme functions at a specific position between two defined amino acids. There are several types of proteolytic enzymes (proteases). Bromelain is a cysteine (sulfhydryl) protease, as are papain from papaya and ficin from figs.

PINEAPPLES

Bromelain is extracted from the pineapple plant. What do pineapples bring to mind? Hawaii? Sun-drenched beaches? A clear, blue sky? Actually pineapples are native to Central and South America. Christopher Columbus is generally credited with their "discovery." During his second voyage to the new world, Columbus landed a shore party on Guadeloupe (in the Caribbean) in 1493. The party promptly got lost but returned several days later with the delicacy we know as pineapple (called "na-na" [meaning fragrance] by the local Carib natives). Columbus sent pineapples back to Europe where its cultivation quickly spread to India, Africa and China. Spanish adventurer Francisco de Paula Marin introduced the fruit to the Sandwich Islands (Hawaii) by the late eighteenth century. But it wasn't until the 1890s that canneries began to preserve this succulent fruit, named because of its resemblance to the pine cone.

Pineapples are one of the most popular tropical fruits. Available year-round, you should consume them fresh, not canned. This is because the heat of canning inactivates the pineapple's enzymes. Have you ever made gelatin? Most packages of gelatin carry a warning to use only canned, not fresh pineapple. The protein-digesting enzymes in the fresh pineapple will break down the gelatin's protein, and it will NEVER gel. Adding fresh pineapple to any food containing any type of protein (such as cottage cheese) will cause changes to occur. These changes, although not harmful, will alter the texture and taste of the finished product.

The pineapple plant grows to two to three feet in height and has sword-shaped, blue-green leaves. The pineapple fruit (at maturity) weighs between four and eight pounds and is supported by a thick stem. It is from this stem that most commercial bromelain is extracted. Although bromelain is present in the plant and the fruit, it is concentrated primarily in the stem before the development of new growth. To extract stem bromelain the outer tissues of the stem are removed and the inner white starchy material is then crushed. The resulting liquid is extracted, filtered, treated, centrifuged, dried and ground.

What is the difference between stem and fruit bromelain? According to research by Fumiko Yamada and colleagues, the two bromelains differ in several ways including molecular weight, isoelectric point, amino acid composition, carbohydrate content (fruit bromelain contains no carbohydrate while stem bromelain has approximately 2 percent), pH optima and specific activity toward protein.[2]

In addition to bromelain, the stem also contains other protease enzymes, including ananain and comosain. According to Takashi Murachi, nonproteolytic enzymes including phosphatase, peroxidase, cellulase and other glycosidases are also present in stem bromelain.[3] Some authors have reported that up to six forms of enzymes can be obtained from stem bromelain.[4]

As a medicine, bromelain is not new. For centuries, fresh pineapple or its stem has been used by South and Central American natives as medicine. Various authors have reported pineapple's ability to improve digestion, quench thirst, act as a diuretic, destroy worms, and treat anorexia, edema, diarrhea and sunstroke. The natives knew pineapple worked wonders and had many healing qualities but they didn't know why. We now know the plant's enzymes are responsible for its varied health-giving activities.

THE POWER OF BROMELAIN

In numerous research studies, bromelain has been shown to:

- enhance and improve digestion;
- fight inflammation (an important factor in injuries, surgeries and numerous conditions);
- keep blood platelets from aggregating (a major cause of strokes, thromboses, heart attacks and other cardiovascular conditions);
- inhibit the growth and spread of cancer (and retard the development of skin cancer caused by exposure to ultraviolet light);
- prevent the attachment of intestinal bacteria infections;
- reduce stress;
- fight many of the effects of aging;
- speed healing from respiratory infections, including sinusitis;
- improve the absorption of drugs, including antibiotics;
- improve the absorption of nutrients, including vitamins;
- improve exfoliation of dead or damaged skin when used topically in cosmetics, facial creams, exfoliants and burn debridement ointments.

HOW TO BUY BROMELAIN

Bromelain can be purchased in individual enzyme form, but is also found in combination with other enzymes (including papain, trypsin, chymotrypsin and pancreatin) to treat many of the above conditions. Bromelain is available without prescription at health food stores, drug and grocery stores, through mail order and multilevel marketing in a variety of forms including:

1. Pills;
2. Tablets;
3. Capsules;
4. Granules;
5. Creams, lotions, gels, ointments and other topical applications.

Be sure to take bromelain with plenty of water. Not only will it help you swallow the pill, tablet or capsule more easily, it also will put the enzyme into solution.

ACTIVITY

Bromelain usually is measured by its weight, in milligrams. Some supplemental bromelain may contain only a few milligrams of the enzyme while others may have as much as 1,200 to 1,500 mg or more. Unfortunately, this does not indicate the strength of the supplement because not all bromelain is the same. Different handling and processing methods may affect the enzyme's potency.

As with every enzyme, bromelain is affected by temperature. Enzyme activity is speeded by heat and slowed by cold. Increased temperatures—such as those used in normal cooking—destroy active enzymes. In fact, temperatures as low as 100°F may destroy some enzymes. Too much heat generated during the processing of bromelain may make the end product weaker than one prepared with less heat.

A good indication of your bromelain's "potency" is the activity level, measured in "units" which should be clearly stated on the label. Bromelain can be measured in many ways including G.D.U. (gelatin dissolving units), M.C.U. (milk clotting units), or F.I.P. (Federation Internationale du Pharmaceutiques) units. Manufacturers themselves sometimes establish their own activity units. For instance, Rhône-Poulenc Rorer Pharmaceuticals, Inc., measures bromelain in "Rorer" units. Unfortunately, these measurement methods are not comparable, nor are they interchangeable. They do offer an excellent way to compare products when the manufacturers use the same unit of measurement, however.

When choosing a bromelain supplement, look for a product that includes at least 600 G.D.U., 900 M.C.U. or 225 F.I.P. per milligram of bromelain.

Bromelain is probably best known for its role in improving digestion, particularly of those foods containing protein. In fact, Columbus' men found that the natives drank pineapple juice to aid digestion (especially when eating meat) and as a bellyache cure.

Our body requires digestive enzymes to assist in breaking down and absorbing nutrients. Proteases digest proteins, amylases digest carbohydrates and lipases digest fats. Deficiencies in these enzymes can cause or lead to bloating, gas, indigestion, candida, food allergies, lethargy, nervous disorders, anemia, osteoporosis and deadly cancer.

The digestive tract is similar to an enclosed assembly line. As food passes through the system it is constantly sprayed and covered by various enzymes (proteases, amylases and lipases), breaking down the proteins, carbohydrates and fats (respectively) in our foods into usable, absorbable particles.

Digestion begins in the mouth as your teeth break up the food into smaller parts, mixing it with saliva. Enzymes in the saliva begin digesting any starches that you eat. To experience the action of saliva on starch, chew a piece of bread, holding it in your mouth for a short time. It will begin to taste sweet because the salivary amylase breaks starch down into maltose (a sugar).

Saliva serves a number of roles. Saliva begins the digestion on starchy foods (such as spaghetti, bread and macaroni), it helps lubricate food for swallowing, helps dissolve solid substances to stimulate the taste buds, cleanses the mouth and teeth (keeping them relatively free of food particles, foreign substances, and sloughed off tissue cells) and helps moisten and lubricate the soft parts of the mouth and lips.

The longer food remains in the mouth, the longer enzymes in the mouth can break up any starches, even before they are swallowed. This is necessary for the breakdown and absorption of foodstuffs into nutrients the body can use.

After swallowing the food, it travels to the stomach where it is broken down into increasingly smaller particles and compounds by various chemical, enzymatic and mechanical means. Hydrochloric acid (HCL) in the stomach helps kill bacteria, improves the absorption of some minerals (such as calcium and iron), and stimulates hormone production. HCL also triggers the conversion of pepsinogen to the active enzyme, pepsin, important in protein digestion. In fact, insufficient hydrochloric acid production (as occurs in achlorhydria and hypochlorhydria) could inhibit the conversion of pepsin from pepsinogen, and protein digestion would suffer. The stomach also produces gastric lipase to split fats, and amylase enzymes to continue carbohydrate digestion. Rennin in the stomach helps release calcium, iron, phosphorus, potassium, and other minerals from milk and other dairy products.

Digestion in the stomach can continue for as long as an hour until food is combined with stomach secretions. This liquid is then emptied into the first part of the small intestine, called the duodenum. The small intestine is composed of three parts: the duodenum, jejunum and ileum. Each division is a vital part of digestion. In fact, the greatest amount of digestion and absorption takes place in the small intestine. In the small intestine, any food solids are reduced to a "paste" called *chyme*.

Triggered by hormones, the gall bladder and pancreas send enzymes necessary for digestion. In addition to its role in insulin and glucagon production, the pancreas also secretes digestive enzymes for all major food types (proteins, carbohydrates and fats). This secretion is rich in at least three proteases as well as amylase and lipase.

The remaining unusable bulk travels from the small to the large intestine (colon) where the job of digestion is completed. The colon contains large numbers of bacteria which produce enzymes that act on the remaining food residues, fiber, cells and mucus discarded from the upper intestinal tract. In the colon, water is absorbed and waste excreted from the rectum as stool.

Enzymes play a decisive role in food breakdown and absorption from the gut to the bloodstream and are essential to the transport of nutrients. If enzyme production or activity is deficient, however, digestion will suffer.

Without adequate digestion good health is impossible. If the digestive system can't adequately break down food for bodily use, even the best dietary intake will be of little value. In addition, without proper breakdown, the body may absorb macromolecules (including whole bacteria). This could lead to infection, intestinal toxemia or irritation, and a number of diseases.

Because bromelain is a protease (that is, it breaks up protein), it can help digest foods containing protein. We need adequate protein in our diet for proper growth, repair, and for the production of antibodies, hormones and enzymes (which themselves are proteins, composed of amino acids).

Bromelain is very helpful in improving digestion because of its wide pH range. We measure acidity or alkalinity on a 15-step scale (0 to 14) known as pH (potential hydrogen). A pH of 7 (water and milk are good examples) is considered neutral (neither acidic nor alkaline), while a high figure (such as 14 for lye) is considered alkaline and a low one (battery acid at 0) is acidic. The mouth has a usual pH range between 6 and 8 (near neutrality).

Characteristically, each enzyme has an optimal pH range which may be broad or narrow. At this "optimum pH" the enzymatic reaction occurs most rapidly. In contrast to the body's digestive enzymes whose pH varies by type and location, bromelain is active through a very wide pH range (3.0 to 8.0) and throughout the entire gastrointestinal tract. Therefore, in those who have a deficiency of digestive enzymes, bromelain can help augment pepsin (an enzyme found in the stomach) and chymotrypsin and trypsin (enzymes in the small intestine).

Bromelain is widely available in digestive products either individually or in combination with other supplements, including enzymes, vitamins, minerals, herbs and other nutrients. When used as a digestive aid, bromelain should be taken from thirty minutes, to just prior to eating a meal. As mentioned, bromelain activity varies; for dosage information follow label instructions. If you don't notice improvement, increase the dose until improved digestion occurs.

THE ISSUE OF ABSORPTION

When bromelain is used to improve digestion it is not necessary that it be absorbed and carried to the bloodstream. This is because all of its activity takes place in the stomach and small intestine. On the other hand, to effectively treat many health conditions it is important that the enzyme be absorbed in the small intestine.

Numerous studies have verified that bromelain (as well as many other enzymes) is absorbed in the small intestine and circulated throughout the body. Although there are several different absorption mechanisms, probably the most frequent mechanism for enzyme absorption is the pinocytotic transfer by the cells of the intestinal wall. *Pinocytosis* is the process by which whole molecules are engulfed and absorbed. After connection to a receptor in the intestinal wall, the enzymes are absorbed, guided through the intestinal cells in vesicles (small sacs), and released into the blood.

Pinocytosis can be compared to taking a hotel elevator from one floor to the next. You walk into the elevator in the lobby and are taken to the second floor. Your body is not broken down into smaller parts but remains intact (whole). Bromelain is transported in much this same way. Approximately 40 percent of bromelain is absorbed intact, thus preserving its enzyme characteristics.

A study by researchers Seifert, Ganser and Brendel measured the amount of bromelain absorbed in adult rats.[5] The bromelain was radioactively labeled and placed directly into the small intestine. Blood and lymph samples were collected during the six-hour observation period and their radioactivity measured. Results show that adult rats can absorb bromelain up to 40 percent in a high molecular form. The researchers noted that this would explain the increased proteolytic activity in serum after bromelain administration, as well as the clinical effect regarding hematoma and edema. This study shows that bromelain, taken orally, can be absorbed from the small intestine into the circulatory system. This absorption is necessary for bromelain to perform its therapeutic activity in the organs and cells of the body.

A randomized, controlled, double-blind study by Castell measured the intestinal absorption of bromelain in humans.[6] A double-blind study is one in which neither the patient nor the investigators has knowledge of which is the active compound and which is the placebo. Bottles are identical and coded. The study included 19 volunteers. Fifteen participants received enteric-coated film tablets containing 200 mg of bromelain while the remaining four individuals received placebo tablets. Blood was collected daily and analyzed for bromelain activity. The researchers found that for most participants, the highest plasma concentration of bromelain was reached at about 48 hours. Researchers concluded that bromelain (taken orally) was found in plasma of human volunteers at clearly measurable concentrations. The bromelain circulating in plasma is apparently not broken down and retains proteolytic activity.

The absorption of bromelain when combined with other enzymes has also been demonstrated. For example, research shows both bromelain and chymotrypsin, taken orally, are absorbed intact from the alimentary tract into the bloodstream.[7,8]

A recent study by I. Donath and colleagues, measured the bioavailability of a mixture containing bromelain and the enzyme, trypsin.[9] In this double-blind, crossover study, the mixture was administered orally four times daily for four days to 21 healthy male volunteers. Blood samples were collected immediately before each dose was given and for two days after the last dose. By using various detection tests, the researchers were able to measure functionally intact bromelain and trypsin in the plasma. Absorption appeared to be dose-dependent.

To clarify the rate of absorption, researchers J. Steffen, J. Menzel and J. Smollen, investigated an enzyme mixture containing bromelain, papain, trypsin, chymotrypsin and pancreatin in guinea pigs.[10] The mixture was given orally to the animals. Tests conducted at 30 minutes, two hours, four hours, and 24 hours after administration showed that the mixture of enzymes was absorbed from the intestine and was present in significant amounts in plasma, urine, heart, kidney, liver and skeletal muscle.

SYSTEMIC ENZYME THERAPY

In addition to its digestive benefits, bromelain is effective in systemic enzyme therapy. This type of therapy—where enzymes travel throughout the system—can maintain wellness, improve health, and fight diseases and injuries. Numerous proteolytic enzymes can be used in this way, each having its own specific properties, advantages and applications. Compared to the enzymes papain, trypsin and chymotrypsin, bromelain seems to have both the greatest effect in reducing swelling and the greatest inhibitory effect on agents which trigger swelling. Because of this, it is helpful in fighting inflammation and inflammatory disorders. In addition, bromelain is effective in inhibiting platelet aggregation (a key cause of cardiovascular disorders) and fighting cancer (by activating tumor necrosis factor). Tumor necrosis factor (TNF) is a type of intercellular mediator, known to attack cancer cells. Bromelain can also help improve the delivery of antibiotics and cancer drugs throughout the body and increase absorption of vitamins and other nutrients.

If you are taking a bromelain supplement for its effectiveness in systemic enzyme therapy, it is important NOT to take it just before or during a meal. Although taking it at this time would serve to improve digestion, to be most effective in systemic enzyme therapy, bromelain should be taken between meals on an empty stomach.

INFLAMMATION

One of the earliest discovered properties of bromelain was its potent anti-inflammatory activity. In fact, the Mayan Indians used fresh pineapples to treat various inflammatory conditions. Today's "medicine men" (and women) know that inflammation plays a critical role in the pathology of many conditions.

If an injury or wound gets hot, red, hurts and swells, it is described as inflammation. Inflammation is an unpleasant, usually painful experience that is a symptom of a number of conditions, including strains, sprains, sinusitis, diabetic ulcers, sore throats, post-operative pain, whiplash pain, back pain and arthritis to name a few. We all encounter one or more of these conditions sometime in our lives.

Viewed biochemically, the history of every acute or chronic inflammation can be divided into three phases. These phases are very gradual and partly overlap, thus preventing any clear-cut demarcation. Inflammation is a dynamic occurrence. The first, initial, phase is the reaction phase (marked by a dilation of the capillaries leading to increased capillary permeability). This stage can last up to 72 hours. The second, or repair phase, typically lasts from 72 hours to six weeks. During this phase, the body continues to eliminate the pathological abnormalities, and attempts to restore normal function. The first condition required is to restore normal circulation to the smallest blood vessels, called the capillaries. Proper circulation helps the body eliminate the highly toxic products resulting from trauma. During the third or regenerative phase (which lasts from three weeks to 12 or more months), the body makes its final effort to correct and repair the damaged tissue. (*See Table 1 next page.*)

The speed at which inflammation occurs and is resolved, is regulated in the body by hormone-like chemicals called *prostaglandins*. Simply put, there are both good and bad prostaglandins in the body. The "bad" prostaglandins stimulate pain receptors, cause pain and encourage inflammation. The "good" prostaglandins decrease the transmission of pain and inhibit inflammation.

The delicate balance that exists between these two groups

TABLE 1
PHASES OF INFLAMMATION

PHASE	DURATION	SYMPTOMS	PHYSIOLOGIC REACTION
Initial *(acute inflammatory or reaction) phase*	Ranges from a few minutes to 72 hours	Swelling, pain, redness, heat, loss of function	Increased capillary (small blood vessel) permeability; plasma flows into the injured area with a build-up of exudate; pre-capillary sphincters constrict and fibrin web is formed at the beginning and end of the damaged area; nutrients and oxygen can't get in and waste products can't get out
Second *(repair)* phase	From 72 hours to 6 weeks	Decrease in swelling, pain, redness and heat; increase in function	Body continues to eliminate the pathological abnormalities; body attempts to restore normal function; improved circulation; decrease of fibrin; collagen is formed
Third (regeneration) phase	From 3 weeks to 12 months or more	Little or no pain, swelling, redness, or heat; return to normal function	Mended area filled-in by connective (scar) tissue and new capillaries (small blood vessels) fibrin is depolymerized by plasmin; proteins are split into peptones and further into amino acids

of prostaglandins (in a healthy body) can be upset when trauma (accident or surgery) or even prolonged stress, occurs. In these situations, the body produces large amounts of "bad" prostaglandins which overwhelm the "good" prostaglandins and prevent the body's defense mechanisms from acting properly. No healing can take place until the original balance is restored.

Technically, stem bromelain is a "selective prostaglandin inhibitor." It decreases the formation of the "bad" prostaglandins and favors those compounds that fight inflammation. According to Steven Taussig, Ph.D., who has done considerable research on the enzyme, bromelain does not affect the "good" prostaglandins whose job is to promote the healing process.[11] In this way, bromelain decreases pain and edema that are part of the inflammatory reaction. By reducing "bad" prostaglandin production to a low level, bromelain reestablishes the normal ratio between the two groups of prostaglandins in the body. This allows the body's own immune system to return to normal.

Acute trauma, such as strains, bruises, sore muscles and minor surgery all involve inflammation. Usually symptoms of these conditions will subside in less than five days when using bromelain.

Bromelain Vs. Apririn and Cortisone

Unlike bromelain, which inhibits only the "bad" prostaglandins, aspirin and other nonsteroidal anti-inflammatory drugs (NSAIDs) completely inhibit *all* prostaglandins. They do this by inhibiting the enzyme, cyclooxgenase—the first step in the inflammatory reaction. Because these drugs have such a broad sweeping effect, however, even the "good" anti-inflammatory prostaglandins are inhibited.

Cortisone is also used to fight inflammation, especially in chronic inflammatory conditions such as arthritis. Cortisone works because it modifies the cell membranes, inhibiting the release of these prostaglandins. During the inflammatory process, however, production of "bad" prostaglandins can increase five- to fiftyfold. By inhibiting their release cortisone allows the "bad" prostaglandins to accumulate in the system because they are not metabolized. This is why cortisone and other corticosteroids can cause such serious side effects.

CIRCULATION

We have seen how bromelain affects the inflammatory reaction and improves recovery time from acute and chronic conditions. Inhibiting excessive clotting of blood provides another example of bromelain's use in health care.

Four to six quarts of blood flow constantly through your blood vessels and are pumped by the heart through the arteries. The arteries gradually narrow into a vast network of capillaries that supply every cell of your body. Some capillaries are so minute that the blood must be squeezed through the cells. After the blood passes through the capillaries, its return trip takes it through larger and larger veins fitted with nonreturn cupped valves. The route back to the heart and lungs is not easy, as the blood must course uphill without much pumping assistance.

There are possibly millions of miles of blood and lymphatic vessels. The size of the vessels in your circulatory system varies from as fine as a microscopic thread to as large as your thumb.

Blood circulates through the heart, arteries, capillaries and veins carrying nutrients and oxygen through the body. It consists of red blood corpuscles (called erythrocytes), a pale yellow liquid (plasma), white blood corpuscles (leukocytes) and thrombocytes—also called blood platelets (disk-shaped objects). The chief role of platelets is blood coagulation.

Blood coagulation is important. Without it, even the smallest injury could cause us to bleed to death. The interaction between liquefaction and coagulation in the blood vessels is one of the most important equilibrium systems in the body.

The body uses a series of inhibitors and activators to control the equilibrum between clot dissolution and formation. In forming a clot, fibrinogen (the plasma protein) is changed to insoluble fibrin (by the enzyme thrombin) and fibrin forms the clot. But fibrin is required by the body for more than just sealing wounds. A continuously thin layer of fibrin also coats the delicate internal blood vessel walls, protecting them from damage. Any small uneven vessel walls are smoothed by fibrin, allowing the blood to flow without creating any disturbances.

To accomplish this, the body produces about two grams of fibrin each day. Without a system of checks and balances, the blood vessel walls could gradually become coated with a thickening layer of this adhesive fibrin. It would become increasingly difficult for blood to flow through the vessels. Finally, blood flow would stop and stasis would follow.

Fortunately, we not only have a system of adhesive fibrin formation but also fibrin dissolution (called fibrinolysis). This system's purpose is to maintain an equilbrium in blood flow by degrading excessive fibrin formation.

The body uses plasmin to break up fibrin protein chains which can be transported away. Unfortunately, the body's plasmin levels decrease with age. At 60, we only possess a fraction of the plasmin that we had when we were young. Therefore, our capacity to break up fibrin is reduced.

This causes an imbalance in the ratio of fibrin to plasmin. Too much fibrin causes the blood to become too thick and sticky. Blood stickiness is a result of insufficient breakdown rate, or fibrin overproduction, and is the most frequent deadly companion of vascular disorders and fatal heart disease. As the flow of blood decreases, toxic debris remains in the vessels and the blood vessels harden and become narrower. Injuries, stress, and other disturbances tend to compound the problem until degenerative symptoms appear (such as insufficient blood flow to the brain or heart, or varicose veins in the legs). Further, individuals with high platelet aggregation values are more susceptible to blood clotting, stroke and heart attack. These conditions frequently appear as we age.

One of the most effective ways of promoting the dissolution of fibrin is through the administration of enzymes, such as bromelain. Bromelain is effective in improving circulatory disorders because it promotes antithrombin activity and prevents blood platelet aggregation.

Research shows bromelain is useful in treating a number of conditions from traumatic disorders (such as injury and surgery) to nontraumatic conditions (including arthritis and sinusitis). These conditions can be acute (of sudden onset) or chronic disorders.

According to *Webster's Dictionary*, chronic means "marked by a long duration or frequent recurrence." So, if you have a disease that is continual or comes and goes but never completely goes away, it is called chronic. Arthritis and cancer are examples of chronic disorders. Chronic disorders and their resulting pain are depressing and highly frustrating to both doctor and patient because modern medicine hasn't unlocked the mystery of their cure.

Two major factors in chronic disorders are inflammation and the immune system. As you now know, acute inflammation is a series of processes (including reaction, repair, and renovation of the damaged area) essential for recovery. Chronic inflammation is more complicated, however, and usually involves some pathological process plus a weakened immune system.

Following are some of the major indications for bromelain's clinical use. This list is in no way all-inclusive, however, as current research is finding new applications for bromelain every day.

AGING

According to the U.S. Census Bureau, by the year 2030 over 21 percent of the American population will be age 65 or older (that figure was just 11 percent in 1980). Unfortunately, the aging process often brings with it increased health problems, including cardiovascular disease, cancer and chronic disorders.

After age 50, the body loses resiliency and various degenerative diseases appear. Hormone secretion diminishes, the production of enzymes decreases, and the immune system is not as effective at fighting off foreign invaders.

As a person ages, his or her enzyme supply decreases in amount and in activity. These decreases are probably at least partially responsible for the development of the characteristic symptoms of aging, and for premature aging. A trivial example of this is provided by the fact that the graying of hair has been attributed to a lack of tyrosinase, or a loss in activity of the enzyme, with advancing age.

To fight illness, most older people take at least one, and often several medications. It is not unusual for a person to be taking one medicine for arthritis, another for high blood pressure, another to help digestion, possibly even sleeping pills and maybe several more drugs if he or she is suffering from cancer.

Most prescription drugs are very potent and can have very serious side effects. In addition, drug reactions can be unpredictable. However, bromelain has many applications for the elderly without serious and long-term side effects. Since bromelain lacks toxicity it appears difficult, if not impossible, to overdose. Bromelain is compatible with, and can be taken with, many drugs.

ARTHRITIS

Any form of arthritis, whether it be osteoarthritis, rheumatoid arthritis or gouty arthritis involves chronic inflammation. To treat this inflammation, physicians prescribe either cortisone or nonsteroidal anti-inflammatory drugs (NSAIDs), such as aspirin and indomethacin. Unfortunately, most drugs used today in the treatment of arthritis can have severe, long-term side effects. For instance, using corticosteroids for a prolonged period of time can lead to cataracts and glaucoma. Even average doses can elevate blood pressure and increase potassium excretion while also increasing the retention of salt and water. Some of the well-known psychic disturbances caused by corticosteroids include insomnia, euphoria, personality changes, mood swings and severe depression.

Fortunately, bromelain can reduce the pain and swelling of arthritis more effectively than drugs and without serious side effects.

A study involving 29 patients (25 with rheumatoid arthritis, one with both osteoarthritis and rheumatoid arthritis, two with osteoarthritis and one with gout) was conducted over a 13-month period.[12] All patients had residual joint swelling and impairment of mobility following long-term corticosteroid therapy. Steroid doses were tapered to small maintenance doses. The patients were given 20 mg tablets of enteric-coated bromelain (four to eight tablets, per day). Each mg was equivalent to 2,500 Rorer units of activity. Swollen joints were measured at the beginning and periodically throughout the study. Results indicated a good to excellent response in 72.4 percent of the cases. In most patients, residual joint swelling was significantly decreased and joint mobility increased soon after bromelain supplementation was initiated. Those taking bromelain had a greater reduction in pain and swelling than those using any other substance. Patients with gouty arthritis experienced poor results, however. There were no harmful side effects detected during or after the test.

According to bromelain authority, Dr. Steven Taussig, bromelain therapy is extremely beneficial as an alternative to NSAIDs and steroidal drugs in the treatment of rheumatoid arthritis.[13] Since these drugs are irritating to the gastrointestinal tract, using bromelain as an alternative can help prevent the onset of gastrointestinal problems.

ATHLETIC INJURIES

Athletes are particularly prone to injuries of all kinds including sprains and strains, skin abrasions, bruises, hematomas (blood-filled bruises), fractures and dislocations. And "weekend warriors" are not immune. In fact, muscles, tendons, ligaments and bones that are not conditioned and not used to constant exercise, are more likely to suffer injury when they are suddenly expected to perform.

One of the best known studies on the use of bromelain with athletes was conducted by J.L. Blonstein in 1969.[14] The double-blind study involved 146 boxers with black eyes and with bruises of the lips, ears, chest or arms. Seventy-four of the boxes received bromelain and 72 received a placebo until the symptoms disappeared. Blonstein found that the black eyes and bruises completely disappeared within four days in 58 of the 74 boxers in the bromelain group. Within the same time frame, only 10 subjects in the placebo group exhibited complete recovery. The bromelain group experienced a more rapid improvement of hematomas and quicker resolution of complaints.

In 1981 a study on 72 soccer players who had suffered muscular strains, sprains and skin abrasions was conducted by P. Mascetti and A. Molteni.[15] The researchers administered bromelain immediately after an injury occurred. Results indicated that 80 percent of the cases had more rapid recovery due to bromelain.

In addition to its anti-inflammatory activity, bromelain can inhibit the formation of blood clots because it has the ability to prevent blood platelets from collecting. This has been demonstrated *in vitro* by Steven Taussig,[16] as well as *in vivo* by R.M. Heinicke.[17] This could be of particular importance for those individuals prone to clotting problems caused by the stress of exercise. One study showed that blood platelet aggregation increased markedly in athletes during a 400 meter race.[18] For this reason, bromelain's ability to inhibit platelet aggregation could be beneficial for athletes.

CANCER

According to the American Cancer Society, "Cancer is a group of diseases characterized by uncontrolled growth and spread of abnormal cells. If the spread is not controlled, it can result in death."[19] Fortunately, major progress has been made in the last few decades to cure many forms of cancer. Researchers are also learning more about how cancer begins, grows and spreads.

The effect of bromelain on various cancer lines has been studied since the early 1970s. In 1972, Guy Gerard (a French physician) first reported the successful use of bromelain in the therapy of breast and ovarian cancers and metastases (cancers that occur when cells from a malignant tumor spread to other areas of the body).[20] The physician used 600 mg of oral bromelain daily from six months to several years in treating 12 patients with breast and ovarian cancer. He reported a marked decrease of most breast cancers and metastases, plus resolution of tumorous masses with ovarian carcinoma. This is a small number of patients, however. Therefore, bromelain's therapeutic effect in this study can only be considered as suggestive and not statistically significant.

According to researchers Lucia Desser and Alexander Rehberger, bromelain stimulates the production of tumor necrosis factor in peripheral blood mononuclear cells of healthy donors.[21] It is also active against cells that have been infected by viruses. One action of the immune system when suffering from infections (whether fungal, viral or bacterial) is to release tumor necrosis factor (TNF).

In a recent issue of *Oncology*, Desser and Rehberger state that bromelain is able to induce TNF, thereby reducing the growth of tumor cells. For this reason, bromelain appears to be an attractive alternative for the treatment of tumors.

High doses of oral bromelain can also taken in combination with subtoxic doses of chemotherapeutic agents such as 5-FU and vincristine. Hans A. Nieper found that this combination, given over a period of four years, resulted in tumor regressions.[22] Neiper hypothesized that bromelain's beneficial action may be due to its "deshielding" of the tumor cell's fibrin coat by fibrinolysis. This action removes the protective fibrin coat surrounding the tumor and allows more ready access to the tumor cells. Now, the immune system can attack the tumor cells directly.

Several researchers have studied bromelain's effect on cancer in mice. Stanley Batkin and his colleagues added bromelain to the diet of mice.[23] They found that bromelain decreased lung metastases of Lewis lung cancer cells implanted beneath the skin in mice. In another study by Batkin, the researchers found that bromelain-supplemented feed decreased the number of metastatic lesions by over 90 percent.[24]

Skin Cancer

One out of every three new cancer cases is skin cancer and one out of every five Americans will develop skin cancer during his or her lifetime. According to the American Cancer Society, almost all of the more than 800,000 cases of squamous and basal cell skin cancer diagnosed each year in this country are sun-related.[19] In fact, the risk from all kinds of skin cancer increases with exposure to sunlight and excessive ultraviolet radiation. A blistering sunburn during childhood can greatly increase your risk of developing melanoma. The link between ultraviolet radiation and skin cancer is so great that laboratory scientists intentionally induce skin cancer in mice by subjecting them to ultraviolet light.

Norman Goldstein and fellow researchers found that bromelain can prevent skin cancer in hairless mice.[25] Researchers gave mice bromelain in their chow at the rate of 80 mg of bromelain for every kg of body weight (a kg is about 2.2 pounds). A second control group of mice received the chow with no bromelain. The mice were then subjected to fifteen minutes of ultraviolet light, three times every week for a period of six months. The first superficial abrasions appeared after two months in the control group but not in the bromelain group.

A subsequent, yet similar study was carried out for twice as long (a full year, rather than just six months) and used 20 mg of bromelain per kg of body weight per day.[26] After one year, all of the control mice (yet only 40 percent of the bromelain group) developed skin cancer. Findings indicate that it took twice as long for the bromelain-fed group to develop lesions as it did for the control group. Apparently, bromelain improves the resistance of animals to the harmful effects of ultraviolet radiation.

CATARACT SURGERY

A cataract is an opaque covering on the eye lens. A common condition of aging, cataracts are the primary cause of blindness worldwide. When cataracts advance to the point where vision is impaired, surgery to remove the crystalline lens of the eye becomes necessary. This improves circulation to the eye.

In 1968, George Spaeth conducted a double-blind study on 111 cataract patients to compare the effect of bromelain to a placebo.[27] Beginning two days before cataract surgery and ending five days after surgery, 59 of the patients received bromelain and the 52 others a placebo. Examinations were conducted daily after the surgery. The author reported that the patients taking bromelain had less swelling of the eyelids and conjunctivae (the membrane that lines the inner eyelid and covers the surface of the eye).

CIRCULATORY DISORDERS

Bromelain appears to prevent blood platelet coagulation, in both *in vivo* and *in vitro* studies.[16,17] This action is extremely significant, since platelet aggregation could be the first step in blood clot formation and narrowing of blood vessels.

In 1972, R.M. Heinicke found that bromelain can prevent blood platelet aggregation.[17] Some of the participants in his study had suffered from myocardial infarctions or strokes within the previous year and all had high platelet aggregation values. Heinicke found that bromelain, taken orally, significantly and rapidly decreased high platelet aggregation values. Formation of a blood clot cannot take place if platelet aggregation does not occur.

The prevention and treatment of cardiovascular disease by bromelain has been discussed earlier in the 1979 study by Steven Taussig and Hans Nieper.[16] Bromelain inhibits platelet aggregation, exerts antianginal activity, relaxes vasoconstriction and promotes fibrinolysis, according to the authors. They feel these actions make bromelain especially useful in treating thrombophlebitis (inflammation of a vein caused by or resulting from a blood clot) and angina pectoris.

In their report, Taussig and Nieper describe bromelain's effect in breaking down cholesterol plaque. The researchers found that, after two hours of taking bromelain in high doses, the blood serum of patients had a potent fibrinolytic activity. That is, the enzyme helped prevent blood platelet aggregation. They also found that bromelain decreases blood pressure in hypertensive subjects to normal levels if administered for an extended period of time.

In a 1962 study, bromelain was given to rabbits in doses as low as 5 mg per kilogram of body weight.[7] R.D. Smyth and his colleagues measured the effect of bromelain on blood clotting parameters (prothrombin time, plasma anti-thrombin levels and serum plasmin concentrations). The animals were given bromelain capsules orally. Blood samples were taken at intervals of one-half, one, one and one-half, two and one-half, three and one-half, four and one-half and sometimes five and one-half hours after the administration of bromelain. The researchers found that bromelain causes an increase in plasmin (which would improve fibrin removal). Again, fibrin is a main component of blood clots. Reducing it reduces the likelihood of abnormal blood clot formation in persons with a tendency to form clots. Elevated antithrombin levels and prolonged prothrombin time seem to prevent fibrin formation. These values remain elevated for two or three hours after taking bromelain. Further, the researchers noted that the dose given to the rabbits was equivalent to a human clinical dose of 350 mg.

The antithrombotic and fibrinolytic action of bromelain may eliminate thrombosis (blood clots) in heart patients. George Felton conducted two large-scale tests on heart patients using bromelain and found practically a complete elimination of thromboses with the enzyme.[28]

Fourteen patients suffering from angina pectoris and coronary heart disease received 1,000 to 1,400 mg of bromelain per day in a study conducted by Dr. Hans Nieper.[29] Symptoms disappeared in all patients taking bromelain within four to 90 days, depending on the severity of coronary scar tissue formation. Further, there were no angina attacks while the patients were taking bromelain. However, when bromelain was discontinued, the angina attacks returned but disappeared as soon as bromelain therapy was again resumed.

The use of oral bromelain in the treatment of acute thrombophlebitis was studied by B. Seligman.[30] Seventy-three patients with acute thrombophlebitis were given bromelain along with painkillers. Results indicated that all symptoms of inflammation improved (pain, redness, edema, tenderness and elevated skin temperature).

At a meeting of the National Heart, Lung and Blood Institute (reported in *Science*, October 1982), the suggestion was made that abnormal blood coagulation might be the body's overall response to cancer, inflammation and heart disease.[31] Therefore, it seems the diseases that respond to bromelain are more interrelated than first thought.

Scientists know that increased fibrin formation seems to be associated with cholesterol and fatty material formation. These, in turn, interfere with circulation. In addition to other circulatory problems this can result in decreased brain, eye, ear, and kidney function as well as heart attacks.

Researcher J.R. Chen conducted *in vivo* and *in vitro* studies of bromelain's effect on cholesterol-protein binding.[32] Results indicated that bromelain broke down arteriosclerotic plaque in rabbit aorta both *in vivo* and *in vitro*.

Bromelain seems to be extremely effective in fighting many circulatory problems. This could include:

- Arteriosclerosis
- Myocardial infarctions
- Thrombosis
- Heart attacks
- Hypertension
- Coronary heart disease
- Thrombophlebitis
- Stroke
- Angina pectoris
- Peripheral venous disease

DENTAL SURGERY

A number of dental procedures require surgery, including tooth extraction, fracture surgery, root canals and abscess removal. Bromelain effectively inhibits inflammation, reduces swelling and decreases pain in dental surgeries.

Gustav Tassman, J.N. Zafran and G.M. Zayon, compared the effectiveness of Ananase (a bromelain product) to a placebo in managing the pain and inflammation that follow oral surgery.[33] All 16 subjects enrolled in the study had a diagnosis of multiple impactions. All except one subject had an impacted third molar. Each patient was given two tablets (either bromelain or a placebo), four times a day beginning 72 hours before surgery and ending 72 hours after surgery. The subjects were examined 24 and 72 hours after surgery. Swelling and pain were evaluated and graded on a scale ranging from "none" to "slight" to "moderate" to "severe." Painkillers were allowed, including salicylates and narcotic analgesics. The researchers found that a greater proportion of the bromelain group were in the "none" and "mild" categories for both inflammation and pain at 24 and 72 hours than those subjects in the placebo group. The differences in distribution were found to be statistically significant.

Another bromelain product (Traumanase) used in dental preprosthetic surgery was evaluated in a study by G. Graber in 1970.[34] The study involving 15 participants was conducted over a three-day period. Participants received two coated tablets of Traumanase four times a day beginning 24 hours before surgery. Bromelain was extremely effective in preventing the development of swelling. By reducing inflammation, fitting the prosthesis was simplified.

DIARRHEA

Diarrhea is a major cause of illness in children. Marked by frequent or watery stools and possible abdominal cramping, it can be particularly dangerous for children because it dehydrates the body and upsets the acid/alkaline ratio. In fact, diarrhea is one of the most frequent causes of acidosis (excessive acidity in the blood), because it rapidly eliminates the alkalizing agents (such as sodium bicarbonate) that are normally found in gastrointestinal secretions. If you have young children, you've probably been cautioned to rush your child to the doctor if prolonged diarrhea should occur. This is because diarrhea can result in severe acidosis which is one of the most common causes of death in young children.

Because of the potentially serious effects of diarrhea, an investigation was conducted by Dr. Tracey Mynott and colleagues to study the possible therapeutic effect of bromelain on bacterial toxins (*Vibrio cholerae* and *Escherichia coli*) which cause diarrhea in humans.[35] Results indicated that bromelain prevents secretion of toxins caused *in vitro* by *Vibrio cholerae* and *Escherichia coli* in rabbit ileum. The researchers concluded that bromelain "may be clinically useful as an antidiarrheal drug."

DIGESTION

Bromelain contains several potent protein-digesting enzymes and has been used for centuries as an aid to digestion and to treat many digestive diseases. For more in-depth information, see the earlier discussion on digestion in this guide.

EPISIOTOMY

An episiotomy is a surgical incision made during childbirth to enlarge the vaginal opening and prevent tearing of these delicate tissues. Though a surgical incision usually heals faster, neater, and with fewer complications than a tear, nevertheless, pain and swelling almost always accompany an episiotomy.

Several studies document bromelain's ability to decrease the pain and swelling that accompany this procedure. In a double-blind, placebo-controlled study, R. Howat and G. Lewis measured the effect of bromelain on episiotomy wounds.[36] The 82 patients in the bromelain group were given two tablets of Ananase (a product containing bromelain) four times per day, while the remaining 70 patients were given a placebo. Researchers measured the development of swelling after surgery, as well as reduction in the bruising. Those taking bromelain experienced more rapid recovery of the wounds than those receiving the placebo.

In another randomized, placebo-controlled, double-blind study conducted by researcher H. Mäder, 99 patients were treated with bromelain, 99 with the painkiller and anti-inflammatory drug, oxyphenbutazone, and 99 with a placebo.[37] Each group received the medication for seven days to measure the effect on episiotomy pain.

Researchers found that those in the placebo group used more painkillers than either the oxyphenbutazone or bromelain groups. Bromelain was as effective as oxyphenbutazone in reducing swelling. According to Mäder, "a high degree of significance could be seen between the results found on the second day after surgery and the third day of treatment." He concluded that bromelain and oxyphenbutazone, in this application, were of equal value.

In the course of a controlled, double-blind study, Gerald Zatuchni and Daniel Columbi treated 160 episiotomy patients with either bromelain or a placebo.[38] Eighty women received the bromelain product Ananase, while 80 received a placebo. Both groups received two tablets, four times daily for three days, beginning four hours after delivery. On the fourth post-operative day, the researchers evaluated any change in inflammation, swelling and pain (at rest and on walking). Body temperature and the amount of narcotics and other painkillers used were also recorded. Results indicated that there were highly significant differences regarding all parameters except temperature, rapidity of ambulation and total days of hospitalization. The bromelain group had substantially less pain at rest and, upon movement, required smaller amounts of painkillers (narcotics), and had lower incidences of infection than the placebo group. It is significant that no adverse effects were observed in any of the patients in the bromelain group.

INFECTIONS

Infections are caused by pathogens, including viruses, bacteria, animal parasites and fungi. The pathogens invade the body either through ingestion (water or food), inhalation (airborne pathogens) or contact (broken skin and animal bites). If not treated promptly and properly, an infection can spread throughout the body and become life-threatening.

Bromelain has been used to fight a number of infections, including bacterial infections (*Escherichia coli*), pneumonia, skin and staph infections, kidney infections, bronchitis and sinusitis (*see* sinusitis later in this book).

Escherichia coli

Escherichia coli (E. coli) is a dangerous bacteria that can cause acute bloody diarrhea in humans. There are several strains of the bacteria, but the one that seems to cause the most trouble in humans is E. coli 0157:H7 which is found naturally in cattle. This bacteria is most often acquired by eating undercooked beef or drinking unpasteurized milk. In October of 1996, however, several cases of E. coli infection were linked to unpasteurized apple juice made from apples that had fallen onto the ground and been contaminated by cow manure.[39] Especially among toddlers in diapers, the organism can also be transmitted from person to person by the fecal-oral route.

According to the Centers for Disease Control and Prevention, infection with E. coli causes approximately 20,000 cases of diarrhea in the United States annually.[40] Approximately 200 deaths are reported every year.

The best way to avoid E. coli is to cook all beef completely, drink only pasteurized milk and juices (unfortunately the pasteurization process also kills most, if not all, of the natural enzymes in the product), wash hands after going to the bathroom and after handling raw meat (especially hamburger), and clean all kitchen utensils thoroughly. It may also be possible to further reduce your risk of acquiring E. coli by using bromelain, as research on rabbits shows.

The virulence of E. coli is due to its ability to adhere to the intestinal wall. If the attachment could be prevented, then the diarrhea that occurs in an E. coli infection could also be prevented.

Researchers recently used bromelain in an attempt to alter the intestinal mucosa and prevent attachment of toxic *Escherichia coli* (ETEC) in rabbits.[41] The study involved forty-four rabbits—half of which received a single oral dose of enterically coated protease granules (a product called Detach containing 25 percent protease). The active ingredient in Detach is bromelain.[42] Eighteen hours later, all the animals were inoculated with different strains of ETEC. Oral administration of the protease preparation containing bromelain decreased diarrhea and diarrhea-caused deaths by 86 percent in the challenged rabbits, while seven of eight (87 percent) of those rabbits not protected by protease (bromelain) treatment developed severe diarrhea or died.

Pneumonia and Other Infections

Two 20-mg enterically coated bromelain tablets were given four times per day to 53 patients suffering from pneumonia, skin and staph infections, kidney infections and bronchitis.[43] The bromelain group also received antibiotics. This sample group was compared to 56 patients who received only antibiotics. Morbidity, judged by the average number of days required for successful treatment, was reduced by more than one-third when antibiotics were supplemented with bromelain. Twenty-three patients who had previously failed to respond to antibiotics improved almost immediately when bromelain was added.

INJURIES (TRAUMAS)

In 1993, over 62 million Americans visited a hospital or doctor's office for treatment of injuries.[44] Sooner or later, each of us will suffer some kind of injury, from a sliver, to a cut, bruise, or bone fracture. Bromelain has been studied extensively and found to be effective in the treatment of injuries, regardless of their cause or type.

The effect of bromelain on 87 patients suffering from various injuries was studied by F. Rühl and H. Otto.[45] Each patient was given four bromelain tablets, four times per day for 14–21 days. Rühl divided the patients into three groups based on the type of injury and came to the following conclusions: The swelling from bruises, contusions and distortions improved within the first two days of therapy. The researcher found minimal improvement in patients who had suffered bruises from fractures, luxations or ligament ruptures, while those patients suffering from inflammatory edemas had a relatively rapid improvement.

Another study measured the effect of bromelain on the swelling, inflammation, sense of heat or tension, and pain resulting from injuries.[46] Participants received two coated tablets of the bromelain product Traumanase every two hours. The dosage was gradually decreased so that, by the fifth day, patients received two coated tablets every four hours. Included in the study were patients suffering from contusions, distortions, fractures, bruises, luxations and general wounds. Sixty-six percent of the cases demonstrated an improvement in the edema (swelling) that occurs after trauma. According to the researcher, a rapid regression of inflammation, swelling, pain, and sense of heat or tension was observed.

Experimental hematomas were induced by Robert Woolf and his colleagues, in the arms and eyelids of volunteers by injecting blood beneath the skin.[47] Participants were given either a bromelain mixture or a placebo (two tablets, four times daily for seven days). According to the researchers, in six out of eight cases, the response of the enzyme group to therapy was considered to be superior. In two cases, no difference was noted between the two series. The researchers concluded that bromelain leads to a more rapid resolution of hematoma of the eyelid and forearm.

MENSTRUAL CRAMPS (DYSMENORRHEA)

The cramping pain most women experience during their monthly menstrual cycle is caused by prostaglandins—the same hormone-like chemicals involved in inflammation. (*See* our discussion on inflammation earlier in this guide.) An excessive amount of these prostaglandins can lead to muscle contractions of the smooth muscles (such as those found in the uterus). Unfortunately, as menstruation approaches, the levels of prostaglandins in a woman's body increase, reaching their height at the onset of the menstrual period. High levels of prostaglandins increase the contractions of the uterus, in turn leading to cramps and pain. These same prostaglandins can escape and find their way into the bloodstream, traveling to other parts of the body and causing headache, diarrhea, nausea, and many other symptoms which accompany menstruation.

One way to reduce menstrual cramps is to reduce the levels of prostaglandins. Many women taken nonsteroidal anti-inflammatory drugs (NSAIDs), such as aspirin and ibuprofen to accomplish this. However, these and other NSAIDs can sometimes cause stomachache, indigestion, diarrhea, nausea and other complications. Several clinical studies have demonstrated the effectiveness of bromelain in reducing menstrual cramping and pain.

Bromelain seems to relax the smooth muscles of the cervix.[48,49] At least in part, this is the reason for bromelain's dramatic effect on the colicky pain noted at the beginning of the period.[49] Bromelain may also decrease the synthesis of those prostaglandins associated with inflammation while increasing levels of compounds which inhibit inflammation.[48]

Twenty-seven patients with dysmenorrhea (painful menstruation due to a hormonal imbalance) and 8 women without menstrual side effects received local applications of bromelain directly on the cervix.[50] The researchers concluded that local bromelain treatment given just before or just after the onset of menstruation results in dramatic relief of pain and associated symptoms for women suffering from primary dysmenorrhea.

Spasmodic dysmenorrhea was studied in thirty patients who had complained of pain which peaked with the onset of menstruation.[49] The patients received local applications of a bromelain solution on the cervix when in pain. Bromelain stopped the cramping pain of spasmodic dysmenorrhea and led to softening of the cervix within a few minutes of application. In some cases, relief continued for as many as four cycles after treatment. The researchers found that the best time to treat with bromelain is shortly before or just at onset of the period.

In another study on dysmenorrhea, researchers measured the effect of a bromelain solution on 64 patients (40 with primary and 24 with secondary dysmenorrhea due to fibroids, tumors or anatomical abnormalities).[51] The patients were treated as soon as cramping accompanied the flow. The bromelain solution was inserted in the vagina and allowed to remain for five minutes. When relief occurred, it was immediate and lasted for the balance of the period. All 40 patients with primary dysmenorrhea had obtained immediate relief. The remaining 24 patients with secondary dysmenorrhea had poor to fair results. The best results occurred with teenagers, women who had never given birth, and a few older patients who had no concurrent gynecologic disease. The success of the younger patients may be because diseases of the cervix are rare in the young.

PLASTIC SURGERY

Plastic surgery builds up tissues, restores a lost or damaged part, or molds a new body part. In these ways, it can be reconstructive, restorative or cosmetic. Unfortunately, plastic surgery can lead to inflammation, swelling, bruising and pain.

A controlled, double-blind study was conducted by Albert Seltzer on 49 patients suffering from swelling due to facial injuries or rhinoplasty (plastic surgery of the nose).[52] Twenty-five patients received the bromelain product Ananase, while 24 received a placebo. Treatment consisted of the necessary surgery, antibiotics, painkillers and ice packs. The only anti-inflammatory tablets were either bromelain or a placebo. Treatment began on the day of the operation. Each patient was given a bottle of 50 tablets of either bromelain or placebo (enough for six days of treatment). When necessary, each patient was given a second bottle and instructed to continue until all the tablets were used. For this reason, treatment varied from between six to twelve days. Results indicated that the ecchymoses (broken blood vessels) and swelling resolved faster than expected in 90 percent of the patients in the bromelain group, but in only 9.5 percent of the placebo group. Seltzer concluded that "bromelains are effective agents for inhibiting the edema and ecchymoses associated with surgical and non-surgical trauma to the face."

A subsequent study on rhinoplasty conducted by P. Baumgartner measured the effect of bromelain on the development of bruises and swelling of the eyelid following surgery.[53] The researcher found that by administering bromelain, the bruises resolved more rapidly, swelling was less extensive (which meant less tension on the suture line) and inflammation resolved more rapidly.

SCLERODERMA

Scleroderma is a condition marked by chronic thickening and hardening of the skin. It may be found in several different diseases and may be localized or appear throughout the systems of the body. It can be characterized by skin thickening and hardening abnormalities involving both the large and small blood vessels, and by degenerative changes marked by the build up of scar tissue in various organs of the body including the lungs, heart, gastrointestinal tract and kidneys.

In one study (reported in the *Journal of Natural Medicine Association*), H. E. Pierce noted that a 32-year-old-woman suffering from scleroderma demonstrated clinical improvement with the use of bromelain therapy.[54] After three months, she was once again able to sleep in a reclining position, clench her fist and eat normal portions of food. Esophageal dysfunction occurs frequently in scleroderma patients. Inflammation of the esophagus and acid reflux are common because the lower esophageal sphincter fails to function properly.

SINUSITIS

Sinusitis is an inflammation of the sinus passages. Common symptoms include pain in the face (especially around the cheeks or eyes), headache and nasal congestion and/or discharge. It is usually caused by an allergic reaction, but can also occur because of viral, fungal or bacterial infections or even injury. Its formation is promoted, for example, through the existence of a septal deviation. The increase in environmental pollutants plays a role in the increasing number of sinusitis cases. In addition, chronic inflammation of the nasal sinuses is frequently the cause of repetitive infections in the lower respiratory tract.

Many people take nasal sprays or use decongestants to help improve drainage and relieve painful symptoms. But bromelain as an adjunctive therapy has been shown effective in speeding recovery from sinusitis.

Back in 1966 S. J. Taub conducted a double-blind, placebo-controlled study on 59 patients suffering from acute or chronic sinusitis to evaluate the effects of bromelain on swelling and inflammation and to measure its effect on nasal discomfort, pain, headaches, generalized ache and breathing difficulties.[55] Participants were given either bromelain or a placebo at the rate of two tablets, four times daily for six days along with either an antibiotic, a decongestant, or both.

Taub found that by the third day of treatment, marked relief of swelling was evident in 55 percent and inflammation in 86 percent of the bromelain group compared to 37 percent and 57 percent, respectively, of the placebo group. Of those receiving bromelain, 66 percent reported relief of breathing difficulties and improvement in nasal discharge, compared to only 40 percent of those in the control group.

In another study, 48 patients suffering from sinusitis

(moderately-severe to severe) were given either bromelain or a placebo for six days after receiving standard sinusitis therapy.[56] Each patient was given two tablets, four times each day. After nine days, the patients were reevaluated. Of those receiving the bromelain, inflammation of the nasal mucosa was completely healed in 83 percent compared to only 52 percent of the placebo group. In addition, 85 percent of the bromelain group found it easier to breathe compared to only 53 percent of those in the placebo group.

SKIN DEBRIDEMENT (BURNS)

Collagen is the main constituent of skin and tendons. A third-degree burn contains collagen in varying stages of denaturation. That in the charred center is completely denatured or destroyed, while fibers around the rim are less denatured and the collagen of the surrounding skin is undenatured. Completely denatured collagen can be decomposed by proteolytic enzymes.

The dead and damaged tissue that remain after a severe burn can contaminate the wound and interfere with proper healing. The surface debris and dead tissue are often anchored to the surface of the wound by strands of collagen. These strands must be broken for debridement to occur. This process is also necessary for prevention of infection. Therefore, physicians "debride" the wound to remove any contaminated, devitalized tissue and foreign material and expose healthy tissue. Debridement can be conducted surgically by actually cutting away the dead or damaged tissue with the aid of chemicals, or by using enzymes which break-up the fibrin, denatured collagen and elastin, but don't destroy the healthy, underlying tissue. By using enzymes, this can provide a clear foundation for skin grafting.

According to J. D. Houck and colleagues, the pineapple stem contains not only proteases (especially bromelain), but also a nonproteolytic segment with contributes to the complete debridement of burns by means of "enzymatic dissection" between the healthy tissue and the burned tissue.[57] The researchers called this enzyme "escharase" and noted that its activity varies enormously from preparation to preparation.

Complete debridement was achieved by P. Klaue, G. Aman and W. Romen on experimental rat burns using 35 percent bromelain in a lipid base.[58] There was no damage to adjacent unburned tissue, and no side effects. Local antimicrobial agents were used at the same time without interfering with bromelain's action. Results from a subsequent study indicated that complete debridement was achieved in 1.9 days.[59] If collagenase (another enzyme used in burn debridement) was used instead of bromelain, however, the debridement period averaged 10.6 days.

Using bromelain permits earlier skin grafting and reduces the risk of infection. In addition, morbidity and mortality of severely burned patients could be significantly decreased with rapid burn debridement.

In addition to burn tissue, bromelain is helpful in the debridement process of removing devitalized tissue from wounds, scars and ulcers.

STRESS

We all have a certain amount of stress in our lives. These stresses can be physical (sports injuries), biochemical (toxic foods) and psychological (divorce and death of a loved one). Some of us can tolerate more stress than others. Regardless of our "tolerance level," however, stress affects our health. When subjected to excessive stress the body produces prostaglandins (as discussed in the section on inflammation). When prostaglandins circulate throughout the body, they cause discomfort because they sensitize pain receptors. These chemicals are produced continuously if stress continues for a long time, leading to digestive problems, chronic degenerative diseases, cancer, ulcers and other conditions.

Bromelain can help return your body to health after periods of stress because it can inhibit production of the "bad" prostaglandins. This will return your body and your health to balance. It can also improve digestion which often suffers during stress.

Scientists have known for at least 35 years that combining bromelain with various antibiotics can improve their effectiveness. Numerous research studies indicate that combining bromelain with an antibiotic (such as tetracycline, penicillin, erythromycin, chloramphenicol, amoxicillin, novobiocin, gentamycin and ampicillin) improves the delivery of the antibiotic to the site of infection, and also makes it possible to use less of the drug to reach the desired effect.[43,60,61,62,63] In Europe, combination drugs such as Traumanase + Tetracycline (by Rorer in Germany) or Enzicyclin (bromelain + tetracycline, by Lepetit in Italy) are frequently used.

In a study by R. Neubauer, over 100 patients suffering from a variety of illnesses, including pneumonia, thrombophlebitis, bronchitis, staph infections, etc., were treated with penicillin, chloramphenicol, erythromycin and novobiocin.[43] Half of the group received the antibiotic only, while the other half received the antibiotic and bromelain. Researchers found that the average number of days required for treatment was reduced by one-third in the bromelain-antibiotic group as compared to the antibiotic-only group. What is especially significant is that 23 of the patients had previously failed to respond to antibiotics. Researchers determined that 90.6 percent of the patients showed excellent or good results from the bromelain-antibiotic mixtures.

S. Tinozzi and A. Vengoni measured the degree to which antibiotic concentration increased with the use of bromelain combined with amoxicillin.[62] The double-blind study involved 42 appendectomy patients, 41 mastectomy patients, and 44 cholecystectomy patients. At the time of measurement, serum levels of the antibiotic were 127 percent higher in the bromelain-antibiotic group than in those receiving just the antibiotic. Antibiotic concentrations were 295 percent greater in the gall bladder and 162 percent greater in bile in the bromelain-antibiotic group.

Another study involved 18 volunteers who were given artificially-induced blisters on each arm.[60] Some of the participants were given bromelain, then after four hours a blood sample was drawn at which time they were then given tetracycline followed by a second dose of bromelain. The second group was given a placebo, then after four hours had blood drawn and was subsequently given tetracycline followed by a second dose of the placebo. Four hours after receiving the tetracycline dose, both groups had another blood sample taken and fluid from the blister was collected. The blisters of the bromelain group contained twice as much tetracycline as the placebo group. The researchers also noted that those in the bromelain group experienced less intense pain at the site of the blister.

Although the above studies were conducted with oral bromelain, it seems to be just as effective when administered by injection. H. Ishikawa and Y. Oguro found that injections of bromelain given before injections of penicillin, gentamycin, or ampicillin in mice infected with *Pseudomonas aeruginosa* (an important causative factor for many infections, including otitis), *Diplococcus pneumoniae* (one cause of pneumonia), or *Streptococcus hemolyticus* (the cause of a variety of respiratory infections), prolonged survival time more than antibiotics alone.[63]

In addition to antibiotics, bromelain can also improve the absorption of cancer chemotherapeutic drugs. This can effectively reduce the amount of the agent needed to treat the tumor without affecting its cancer-fighting abilities. Drugs used in cancer therapy are highly cytotoxic, so the ability to use less drug and still maintain the same effect is particularly important in enhancing the life of the cancer patient.

IMPROVING ABSORPTION OF OTHER NUTRIENTS

According to bromelain expert Steven Taussig, it is possible that bromelain improves the absorption of most active ingredients in common foods, such as vitamins and other essential nutrients. Many vitamin, mineral, and herbal manufacturers combine bromelain with other nutrients since the enzyme improves the digestion, absorption and bioavailability of these nutrients.

In addition, combining bromelain with vitamins, minerals and other nutrients is an excellent way to further improve your health. Most commonly recommended are vitamins A, B complex, C, and E, and such minerals as selenium, zinc and magnesium. The dosages and particular combinations, however, go beyond the scope of this guide. Nevertheless, the dosages of vitamins and minerals must be determined individually with attention being paid to the clinical picture, the therapy, as well as the constitution of the individual.

DOSAGE

The amount of bromelain needed for any condition will vary depending on several factors:

1. The activity (potency) of the bromelain product.

2. The condition being treated.
3. Your height and weight.
4. Your health status.
5. Your age.

Because of the above variables, the amount of bromelain needed to treat any specific condition can vary widely between individuals. The above studies can serve as guidelines; however, a good baseline dosage with which to begin might be three to four 230 to 250 mg capsules or tablets per day. In general, acute injuries will respond more quickly than chronic disorders. With an acute injury, if no response is noted within three days, increase the dosage until you see symptom improvement. On the other hand, chronic disorders, such as rheumatoid arthritis might require four to six weeks before improvement is noted. Although no immediate change will be noted, it is important to continue the enzyme therapy.

BROMELAIN IN ENZYME COMBINATIONS

As an individual enzyme, bromelain is extremely effective for specific conditions. However, bromelain has also been used in combination with other enzymes such as papain, pancreatin, trypsin, chymotrypsin and microbial enzymes, as well as other nutrients, including the bioflavonoid, rutin.

There are many advantages to using a combination of enzymes over an individual enzyme. Enzymes work at certain acidity or alkalinity levels and temperatures, which differ from enzyme to enzyme. By having enzymes from a wide variety of origins (plant, fungi, animal) more areas in the body will be treated. There can be a synergism of the combined enzymes, increased percentage of absorption, increased level of effectiveness and broader range of application.

Bromelain, or bromelain in combination with other enzymes, has a wide range of proven applications:

1. Digestive disorders, including indigestion, gas, constipation, diverticulitis and diarrhea.
2. Circulatory disorders, including pathological venous disorders, post-thrombotic syndrome, occlusive arterial disease, thromboembolic complications and lymphedema.
3. Inflammation in general, including acute and chronic bronchitis, sinusitis, prostatitis, cystitis, cystopyelitis and pelvic inflammatory disease.
4. Rheumatic diseases including rheumatoid arthritis (chronic polyarthritis), ankylosing spondylitis (Bechterew's disease), soft tissue rheumatism including myositis, polymyositis, polychondritis, tendosynovitis, synovitis, tendonitis, tennis elbow, bursitis, non-articular rheumatic syndrome, and degenerative rheumatism conditions, including joint disease and monoarticular active osteoarthrosis.
5. Surgery, including operative dentistry, proctology and bypass surgery.
6. Traumatology, including operative treatment, fracture reduction, meniscectomy, arthroscopic meniscectomy, sprained ankles, soft tissue injuries and absorption of hematomas.
7. Cancer therapy (including breast, prostatic, lung, brain, pancreatic, colorectal and uterine).
8. Sports injuries, including therapy and prevention.
9. Viral disorders such as herpes zoster, herpes simplex and HIV infections.
10. Other disorders including fibrocystic breast disease, multiple sclerosis, ulcerative colitis (Crohn's disease) and pancreatitis.

SIDE EFFECTS AND SAFETY ISSUES

Currently, bromelain is classified as a food or food ingredient which is "generally recognized as safe" (GRAS). Although rare, reactions to bromelain could occur and might include diarrhea, nausea, vomiting and skin sensitivities. Simply cutting back on the dose will alleviate these symptoms. According to Steven Taussig, bromelain is nontoxic and no harmful side effects have occurred even at doses ten to twenty times higher than normally recommended.

There are, however, contraindications. Because bromelain improves blood fluidity (which is why it is so helpful in cardiovascular problems), this can present problems for individuals suffering from hemophilia or those on anti-coagulant medications whose blood may already be very thin and lack coagulation factors.

CONCLUSION

Bromelain is a health-giving enzyme from the tropical forests. Yes, it's bromelain—bursting from the nutritious pineapple stem. Bromelain—a cherished healer, a gift of health and life from our ancestors:

- improves digestion;
- is a potent anti-inflammatory agent that acts on a wide variety of disorders, including bruises, strains, rheumatoid arthritis, ulcers and edema;
- prevents clumping of blood platelets (a primary cause of stroke, thrombosis and heart attack);
- prevents the growth and spread (metastasis) of cancer cells and significantly retards development of skin cancer (caused by ultraviolet light);
- speeds healing from surgery;
- improves absorption of nutrients and drugs;
- fights and results of aging;
- decreases wrinkles and removes dead skin from face and body (when used topically as an exfoliant);
- removes devitalized tissue from burn injuries.

Bromelain is effective individually or in combination with other enzymes. It has no side effects of long-term duration. It causes no toxic build-up in the body. Therefore, bromelain can be effectively used for extended periods of time.

Since bromelain has a wide range of applications, companies and research institutions are beginning to test bromelain for expanded uses such as immune and autoimmune disorders and HIV/AIDS. In addition, they are analyzing bromelain's ability to increase the potential for certain medications.

For further information on enzymes, see my other enzyme books, *Enzymes and Enzyme Therapy: How to Jump Start Your Way to Lifelong Good Health* and *Enzymes: Nature's Energizers* published by Keats Publishing, Inc.

REFERENCES

1. Dalling, Michael J. *Plant Proteolytic Enzymes.* Vol. I (Boca Raton: CRC Press, Inc., 1986), 86.
2. Yamada Fumiko, Takahashi Noriko, Murachi Takashi. 1976. "Purification and characterization of a proteinase from pineapple fruit, fruit bromelain FA2." *J. Biochem.* 79:1223–1234.
3. Murachi, Takashi. 1976. "Bromelain Enzymes." *Methods in Enzymology.* 45:475–485.
4. Ota Shoshi, Muta Eiko, Katahari Yasuko, Okamoto Yoshiko. 1985. "Reinvestigation of fractionation and some properties of the proteolytically active components of stem and fruit bromelains." *J. Biochem.* 98:219–228.
5. Seifert J., Ganser R., Brendel W. "Die Resorption eines Proteolytischen Enzyms Pflanzlichen Ursprungs aus dem Magen-Darm-Trakt in das Blut und die Lymphe von erwachsenen Ratten." *Z. Gastroenterol.* 17(1):1–8 (January, 1979).
6. Castell, J.V. "Intestinal absorption of undegraded bromelain in humans," in: M.L.G. Gardner and K.-J. Steffens (eds.), *Absorption of Orally Administered Enzymes* (Berlin: Springer Verlag, 1995), 47–60.
7. Smyth R.D., Brennan Rita, Martin Gustav J. 1962. "Systemic biochemical changes following the oral administration of a proteolytic enzyme, bromelain." *Arch. Int. Pharmacodyn.* 136(1–2):230–236.
8. Kabacoff B.L., Wohlmann A., Umhey M., Avakian S. 1963. "Absorption of chymotrypsin from the intestinal tract." *Nature.* 199:815.
9. Donath I., Mai A., Maurer A., Brockmöller J., Kuhn C.-S., Friedrich G., Roots I. 1997. "Dose related bioavailability of bromelain and trypsin after repeated oral administration." *Clin. Pharm. & Therap.* 61(2):157.
10. Steffen J., Menzel J., Smolen J. 1979. "Untersuchungen über intestinale

resorption mit 3H-markiertem Enzymgemisch." *Acta Med. Austriaca.* 6:13–18.

11. Taussig, Steven. 1980. "The mechanism of the physiological action of bromelain." *Med. Hypotheses.* 6:99–104.
12. Cohen, A., Goldman, J. "Bromelain therapy in rheumatoid arthritis." *Penn. Med. Jnl.* 67:27–30 (June 1964).
13. Taussig, personal communication with author. August 5, 1997.
14. Blonstein, J.L. "Control of swelling in boxing injuries." *Practitioner.* 203:206 (August, 1969).
15. Mascetti, P., Molteni, A. 1981. "Enzimi proteolitici mucopiolitici in associazione nella medicina sportiva." *Med. Sport.* 34:399–402.
16. Taussig, Steven J., Nieper, Hans A. 1979. "Bromelain: Its use in prevention and treatment of cardiovascular disease: present status." *Journal of IAPM.* VI(1):139–150.
17. Heinicke, R.M., van der Wal, Linda, Yokoyama, M. 1972. "Effect of bromelain (Ananase) on human platelet aggregation." *Experientia.* 28:844–845.
18. Leuscher, E.F. "Effect of various agents on platelet function: platelets vessel wall-fibrin." *Deposition Symp. 1969* (Stuttgart: Georg Thieme, 1970), 41–52.
19. American Cancer Society, *Cancer Facts & Figures–1996* (Atlanta: American Cancer Society, Inc., 1996).
20. Gerard, Guy. 1972. "Therapeutique anti-cancreuse et bromelaines." *Agressologie.* 3:(4)261–274.
21. Desser, Lucia, Rehberger, Alexander. 1990. "Induction of tumor necrosis factor in human peripheral-blood mononuclear cells by proteolytic enzymes." *Oncology.* 47:475–477.
22. Nieper, Hans A. 1976. "Bromelain in der kontrolle malignen washstums." *Krebsgeschehen.* 1:9–15.
23. Batkin, Stanley, Taussig, S.J., Szekerez, J. 1988. "Antimetastatic effect of bromelain with or without its proteolytic and anticoatgulant activity." *J. Cancer Res. Clin Oncol.* 114(5):507–508.
24. Batkin, Stanley, et al. 1988. "Modulation of pulmonary metastasis (Lewis lung carcinomas) by bromelain, an extract of the pineapple stem (Ananas comosus), Letter., *Cancer Invest.* 6(2):241–242.
25. Goldstein, Norman, Taussig, Steven J., Gallup, James D., Koto, Vernon. "Bromelain as a skin cancer preventive in hairless mice." *Hawaii Medical Journal.* 34(3): 91–94 (March, 1975).
26. Taussig, Steven, Goldstein, Norman. 1976. "Effect of bromelain on cancer." *Krebsgeschehen.* 8(4):81–87.
27. Spaeth, George L. "The effect of bromelains on the inflammatory response caused by cataract extraction: A double-blind study." *Eye, Ear, Nose, Thr. Monthly.* 47(12):634–639(December, 1968).
28. Felton, George E. "Fibrinolytic and antithrombotic action of bromelain may eliminate thrombosis in heart patients." *Medical Hypothesis.* 6(11):1123–1133 (November, 1980).
29. Nieper, Hans. 1978. "Effect of bromelain on coronary heart disease and angina pectoris." *Acta Med. Empirica.* 5:274–275.

30. Seligman, B. 1969. "Oral bromelains as adjuncts in the treatment of acute thrombophlebitis:" *Angiology.* 20:22–26.
31. Marx, J.L. 1982. "Coagulation as a common thread in disease." *Science.* 218:145–146.
32. Chen, J.R. 1975. "In vivo and in vitro studies of the effect of bromelain on cholesterol-protein binding." *Dissert. Abstr.* B 35 (2 pt), 6013, Ord. No. 75-13, 735.
33. Tassman, Gustav C., Zafran, J.N., Zayon, G.M. 1965. "A double-blind crossover study of a plant proteolytic enzyme in oral surgery." *J. Dent. Med.* 20:51–54.
34. Graber, G. 1970. "Klinische Erfahrungen mit dem pflanzlichen proteolytischen Enzymkomplex Traumanase in der zhanärztlichen präpropthetischen Chirurgie." *Schweiz, Zahnheilk.* 80:1206–1212.
35. Mynott, Tracey L., Guandalini, S., Raimondi, F., Frasano, A. "Bromelain prevents secretion caused by Vibrio cholerae and Escherichia coli enterotoxins in rabbit ileum in vitro." *Gastroenterology.* 113(1):175–184. (July, 1997).
36. Howat, R.C.L., Lewis, G.D. "The effect of bromelain therapy on episiotomy wounds—a double-blind controlled clinical trial." *J. Obstet. Gynaec.* 79:951–953 (October, 1972).
37. Mäder, H. 1973. "Vergleichende untersuchung zwischen Bromelain und Oxyphenbutazon auf ihre Wirkung bei Episiotomie-Schmerzen." *Schweiz. Rdsch. Med. Prax.* 62:1062–1067.
38. Zatuchni, Gerald I., Colombi, Daniel J. "Bromelain therapy for the prevention of episiotomy pain." *Obst. Gynecol.* 29(2):275–278 (February, 1967).
39. *Morbidity and Mortality Weekly Report.* "Outbreaks of Escherichia coli O157:H7 infection and cryptosporidiosis associated with drinking unpasteurized apple cider—Connecticut and New York." 46(1) (January 10, 1997).
40. *Morbidity and Mortality Weekly Report.* "Enhanced detection of sporadic Escherichia coli O157:H7 infections—New Jersey, July 1994." 44(22) (June 9, 1995).
41. Mynott, Tracey, Chandler, David S., Luke, Richard K.J. "Efficacy of enteric-coated protease in preventing attachment of enterotoxigenic Escherichia coli and diarrheal disease in the RITARD model." *Infection and Immunity.* 59(10):3708–3714 (October, 1991).
42. Mynott, L., personal communication with author, July 2, 1997.
43. Neubauer, R. 1961. "A plant protease for the potentiation of and possible replacement of antibiotics." *Exp. Med. Surg.* 19:143–160.
44. *Statistical Abstract of the United States; 1995.* 115th edition. (Washington, D.C.: U.S. Bureau of the Census, 1995), 138.
45. Rühl, F., Otto, H. 1965. "Über die perorale Therapie posttraumatischer Schwellungen und Hämatome mit dem pflanzlichen, proteolytischen Ferment Bromelain." *Therapiewoche.* 11:555–559.
46. Bünnagel, W. 1966. "Erfahrungen mit einem proteolytischen Enzym in der Landpraxis." *Therapiewoche.* 35:1163–1164.
47. Woolf, Robert M., Snow, John W., Walker, J. Harris, Broadbent, T.

Ray. 1965. "Resolution of an artifically induced hematoma and the influence of a proteolytic enzyme." *J. Trauma.* 5:491–494.

48. Felton, George E. "Does kinin release by pineapple stem bromelain stimulate production of prostaglandin E1-like compounds?" *Hawaii Med. Jnl.* 36(2):39–47. (February 1977).

49. Simmons, Clifford. "The relief of pain in spasmodic dysmenorrhea by bromelain." *Lancet.* 827–830 (October 28, 1958).

50. Youssef, A.H. 1960. "The uterine isthmus and its sphincter mechanism: a clinical and radiographic study. III. The effect of bromelain on the uterine isthmus." *Am. Jnl. Obstet. Gynecol.* 79(6):1161–1168.

51. Hunter, Robert G., Henry, George W., Heinicke, R.M. "The action of papain and bromelain on the uterus." *Am. Jnl. Obstet. Gynecol.* 73(4):867–874 (April, 1957).

52. Seltzer, Albert P. 1964. "A double-blind study of bromelain in the treatment of edema and ecchymoses following surgical and nonsurgical trauma to the face." *Eye, Ear, Nose, Thr. Monthly.* 43:54–57.

53. Baumgartner, P. 1970. "Erfahrungen mit Tramanase bei postoperativen Hämatomen." *Praxis.* 59:217–219.

54. Pierce, H.E. 1964. "Pineapple proteases in the treatment of scleroderma—a case report." *Jnl. Natl. Med. Assoc.* 56(3):272–273.

55. Taub, S.J. 1966. "The use of Ananase in sinusitis: A study of 60 patients." *Eye, Ear, Nose, Thr. Monthly.* 45:96, 98; also, "The use of Bromelains in sinusitis: a double-blind clinical evaluaton."*Eye, Ear, Nose, Thr. Monthly.* 46(3):361–365 (March, 1967).

56. Ryan, R.E. 1967. "A double-blind clinical evaluation of bromelain in the treatment of acute sinusitis." *Headache.* 7(1):13–17.

57. Houck, J.D., Chang, C.M., Klein, G. 1983. "Isolation of an effective debriding agent from the stems of pineapple plants." *International Journal of Tissue Reactions.* 2:125–135.

58. Klaue, P., Aman, G., Romen, W. 1979. "Chemical debridement of the burn eschar in rats with bromelain combined with topical antimicrobial agents." *European Surgical Research.* 355–359.

59. Klaue, P., Dilbert, G., Hinke, G., Schmelzer, V., Romen, W. 1979. "Tier-Experimentelle Untersuchungen zur enzymatischen Lokalbehandlung Subdermaler Verbrennungen mit Bromelain." *Therapiewoche.* 29:796–799.

60. Bodi, T. 1965. "Modification of tissue permeability by oral bromelain in man." *Expt. Med. Surg. Suppl.* 51–56.

61. Renzini, G. 1972. "The absorption of tetracyclin in presence of bromelains during oral application." *Drug Research.* 22:410–412.

62. Tinozzi, S., Vengoni, A. 1978. "Effect of bromelain on serum and tissue levels of amoxycillin." *Drugs Under Experimental and Clinical Research.* 4:39–44.

63. Ishikawa, H., Oguro, Y. 1974. Green Cross Research Laboratory, Osaka, Japan, in *Jap. Journ. Antibiot.* 27(2), 118–121.

Manufacturer or Distributor

Amano Enzyme U.S.A. Co., Ltd.
1157 North Main Street
Lombard, Illinois 60148
Tel: (800) 446-7652
Fax: (630) 953-1895

American Biologics
1180 Walnut Avenue
Chula Vista, California 91911
Tel: (619) 429-8200
Fax: (619) 429-8004

American Dietary Labs
14631 Best Avenue
Norwalk, California 90650
Tel: (800) 423-8837

American Laboratories, Inc.
4410 S. 102nd St.
Omaha, Nebraska 68127
Tel: (800) 445-5989
Fax: (402) 339-0801

Anabolic Laboratories, Inc.
17801 Gillette Avenue
P.O. Box C19508
Irvine, California 92713
Tel: (714) 863-0340
Fax: (714) 261-2928

Apex Energetics
1701 E. Edinger Ave., A-4
Santa Ana, CA 92705
Tel: (800) 736-4381

Ashland Nutritional Products
17751 Mitchell
Irvine, California 92714
Tel: (714) 833-9500
Fax: (714) 833-9595

Biotics Research Corporation
P.O. Box 36888

Houston, Texas 77236
Tel: (713) 240-8010

CC International, Inc.
P.O. Box 2452
Rancho Santa Fe, California 92067
Tel: (800) 775-3575
Fax: (619) 756-1334

Crystal Star Herbal Nutrition
250 Country Club Heights
Carmel Valley, California 93924
Tel: (800) 532-6015
Fax: (408) 659-7640

Douglas Laboratories, Inc.
600 Boyce Road
Pittsburgh, Pennsylvania 15205
Tel: (888) DOUGLAB
Fax: (412) 494-0155

Energetica Natura Benelux BV
Baudeloo 20A
4561 ES Hulst, The Netherlands
Tel: +31/114-321-461
Fax: +31/114-319-397

Enzymatic Therapy, Inc.
825 Challenger Drive
Green Bay, Wisconsin 54311
Tel: (800) 558-7372
Fax: (414) 469-4400
http://www.enz.com

Enzyme Development Corporation
2 Penn Plaza, Suite 2439
New York, New York 10121-0034
Tel: (212) 736-1580
Fax: (212) 279-0056

Enzyme Process International
2035 E. Cedar Street
Tempe, Arizona 85281

Tel: (800) 521-8669
Fax: (602) 731-9432

Futurebiotics, Inc.
145 Ricefield Lane
Hauppauge, New York 11788
Tel: (516) 273-6300
Fax: (516) 273-1165

Garden State Nutritionals
100 Lehigh Drive
Fairfield, New Jersey 07004
Tel: (800) 526-9095
Fax: (201) 575-6782

General Nutrition, Inc.
921 Penn Avenue
Pittsburgh, Pennsylvania 15222
Tel: (412) 288-4713

General Research Laboratories
8900 Winnetka Avenue
North Ridge, California 91324
Tel: (800) 421-1856
Fax: (818) 407-8500

Gero Vita
6021 Yonge Street
Toronto, Ontario, Canada M2M 3W2
Tel: (800) 694-8366

HealthSmart Vitamins
1921 Miller Drive
Longmont, Colorado 80501
Tel: (800) 492-3003

Herbal Products and Development
P.O. Box 1084
Aptos, California 95001
Tel: (408) 688-8706
Fax: (408) 688-8711

Highland Laboratories
110 South Garfield
Mt. Angel, Oregon 97362
Tel: (800) 547-0273

Interior Design Nutritionals
75 West Center Street
Provo, Utah 84601
Tel: (801) 345-2000
Fax: (801) 345-1999

KAL, Inc.
P.O. Box 4023
Woodland Hills, California 91365
Tel: (818) 340-3035

K.-W. Pfannenschmidt GmbH.
P.O. Box 610151
22421 Hamburg, Germany
or
Habichthorst 36
22459 Hamburg, Germany
Tel: (040) 555-866-0
Fax: (040) 555-3898

Life Plus
P.O. Box 3749
Batesville, Arkansas 72503
Tel: (800) 572-8446

Marcor Development Corp.
108 John Street
Hackensack, New Jersey 07601
Tel: (201) 489-5700
Fax: (201) 489-7357

Michael's Naturopathic Programs
6820 Alamo Downs Parkway
San Antonio, Texas 78238
Tel: (210) 647-4700

Mucos Pharma GmbH & Co.
Malvenweg 2
D-82538 Geretsried
Germany
Tel: (+49) 0 8171 5180
Fax: (+49) 0 8171 52008

National Enzyme Company
P.O. Box 128
Forsyth, Missouri 65653
Tel: (800) 433-8589
Fax: (417) 546-6433

Natrol, Inc.
20731 Marilla Street
Chatsworth, California 91311
Tel: (800) 326-1520
Fax: (818) 701-0623

Naturally Vitamin Supplements Co.
14851 N. Scottsdale Road
Scottsdale, Arizona 85254
Tel: (800) 899-4499
Fax: (602) 991-0551

Nature's Life
7180 Lampson Avenue
Garden Grove, California 92841
Tel: (714) 379-6500
Fax: (714) 379-6501

Nature's Plus
548 Broad Hollow Road
Melville, New York 11747

Tel: (516) 293-0030
Fax: (516) 249-2022

Now Foods
550 Mitchell
Glendale Heights, Illinois 60139
Tel: (800) 999-8069

Nutri-West
P.O. Box 950
Douglas, Wyoming 82633
Tel: (307) 358-5066

Oekpharma GmbH
Moosham 29
A-5580 Unternberg, Austria
Tel: +43-6476-805-0
Fax: +43-6476-805-40

PhysioLogics
6565 Odell Place
Boulder, Colorado 80301-3330
Tel: (800) 765-6775

PhytoPharmica
825 Challenger Drive
Green Bay, Wisconsin 54311
Tel: (800) 553-2370
Fax: (414) 469-4418

Phyto-Therapy, Inc.
P.O. Box 555
Franklin Lakes, New Jersey 07417
Tel: (201) 891-1104
Fax: (201) 848-1867

Professional Health Products
P.O. Box 80085
Portland, OR 97280-1085
Tel: (800) 952-2219
Fax: (503) 452-1239

Progressive Laboratories, Inc.
1701 W. Walnut Hill Lane
Irving, Texas 75038
Tel: (214) 518-9660
Fax: (214) 518-9665

Quad Laboratories
P.O. Box 555
Franklin Lakes, New Jersey 07417
Tel: (201) 891-1104
Fax: (201) 848-1867

Rainbow Light Nutritional Systems
P.O. Box 600
Santa Cruz, California 95061
Tel: (800) 635-1233

Schiff Products, Inc.
1960 South 4250 West
Salt Lake City, Utah 84104
Tel: (801) 975-5000
Fax: (801) 972-6532

Solgar Vitamin and Herb Co.
500 Willow Tree Road
Leonia, New Jersey 07605
Tel: (800) 645-2246
Fax: (201) 944-7351

Specialty Enzymes and Biochemicals Co.
5390 La Crescenta
Yorba Linda, California 92687
Tel: (714) 692-3350
Fax: (714) 692-3051

Triarco, Inc.
6 Morris Street
Paterson, New Jersey 07501
Tel: (201) 278-7300
Fax: (201) 278-0317

Twin Laboratories, Inc.
2120 Smithtown Avenue
Ronkonkoma, New York 11779
Tel: (516) 467-3140
Fax: (516) 471-2375

Tyler Encapsulations
2204 N.W. Birdsdale
Gresham, Oregon 97030
Tel: (503) 661-5401
Tel: (800) 869-9705

Vitagenics
240 South Broad St.
P.O. Box 886
Elkhorn, Wisconsin 53121
Tel: (414) 723-4942
Fax: (414) 723-5462

Vitamin Research Products, Inc.
3579 Highway 50 East
Carson City, Nevada 89701
Tel: (800) 877-2447
Fax: (702) 844-1331

Wild Rose Herbal Formulas
#203, 8173-128th St.
Surrey, B.C. V3W 4G1
Canada
Tel: (604) 591-8881
Fax: (604) 597-1784

.